Can I tell you about Diabetes (Type 1)?

Can I tell you about...?

The "Can I tell you about...?" series offers simple introductions to a range of limiting conditions and other issues that affect our lives. Friendly characters invite readers to learn about their experiences, the challenges they face and how they would like to be helped and supported. These books serve as excellent starting points for family and classroom discussions.

Other subjects covered in the "Can I tell you about...?" series

ADHD

Adoption

Asperger Syndrome

Asthma

Cerebral Palsy

Dementia

Dyslexia

Epilepsy

ME/Chronic Fatigue Syndrome

OCD

Parkinson's Disease

Selective Mutism

Stammering/Stuttering

Tourette Syndrome

Can I tell you about Diabetes (Type 1)?

A guide for friends, family and professionals

JULIE EDGE

Illustrated by Julia MacConville

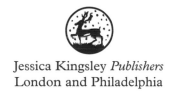

Jessica Kingsley *Publishers*
London and Philadelphia

First published in 2014
by Jessica Kingsley Publishers
73 Collier Street
London N1 9BE, UK
and
400 Market Street, Suite 400
Philadelphia, PA 19106, USA

www.jkp.com

Library of Congress Cataloging in Publication Data
Edge, Julie, author.
Can I tell you about diabetes (type 1)? : a guide for friends, family
and professionals / Julie Edge ; illustrated by Julia MacConville.
pages cm. -- (Can I tell you about--?)
Audience: Ages 7+.
Includes bibliographical references.
ISBN 978-1-84905-469-0 (alk. paper)
1. Diabetes in children--Juvenile literature. I. MacConville, Julia,
illustrator. II. Title. III. Series: Can I tell you about-- ? series.
RJ420.D5E34 2014
618.92'462--dc23
2013048185

British Library Cataloguing in Publication Data
A CIP catalogue record for this book is available from the British Library

ISBN 978 1 84905 469 0
eISBN 978 0 85700 845 9

Printed and bound in Great Britain by Bell & Bain Ltd, Glasgow

This book is dedicated to all the children
with diabetes and their families with
whom I have had the pleasure of working
with during my 26 years in Oxford.

Acknowledgements

I would like to thank Lucy Buckroyd for offering me the opportunity to write this book to add to the "Can I tell you about...?" series.

I would also like to thank Julia MacConville for capturing the character of Debbie just perfectly in her delightful illustrations.

Thanks also go to all the people I have worked with over the years, who have taught me all I know about diabetes, including the children, young people and their families. Thanks particularly to Jane Haest for her very helpful comments on the book.

Finally, I would like to thank my wonderful family for all their patience and support.

Contents

Introduction

This book aims to help children and young people from seven years upwards and their friends and family and professionals gain a clearer understanding of type 1 diabetes.

- It will describe what this type of diabetes is, explain what it feels like to have diabetes, how other people treat you and what to do in an emergency. It will also discuss what happens at the diagnosis of diabetes and the things that a family will need to learn.

- It is a useful aid to prompt discussion both in the classroom and at home.

- Many teachers and parents are already very aware of diabetes and how they can help. For those teachers and parents, this book should act as a refresher and a means of support. The two extra sections at the back of the book offer tips for how teachers and parents can help children with diabetes.

- Type 1 diabetes is one kind of diabetes, and is the commonest form in children: 97 per cent of children with diabetes in the UK have type 1. To make this book easier to read I have used diabetes for short throughout, except where a distinction from other types is important.

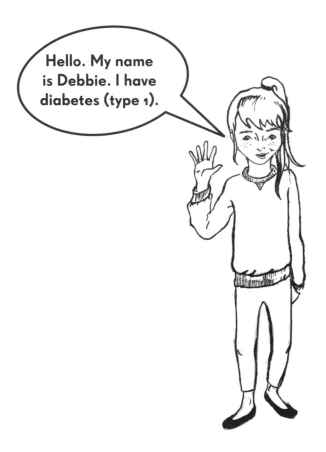

"I'd like to tell you what it's like to have diabetes."

"My name is Debbie and I have type 1 diabetes. (I will call it diabetes from now on but I'll be talking about type 1.)

I have had it since I was six years old and no one in my family has it, so sometimes it makes me feel very lonely. You can't tell by looking at me that I have diabetes and I can do everything that everyone else my age can do, but I need to do a bit more planning ahead.

When I was much younger I didn't understand anything about my diabetes. My parents have helped me to manage my diabetes every day since I've had it and I am now learning about it myself so that I can do the same things as my friends and can go round to their houses for sleepovers.

Diabetes means that I have to be careful about what I eat. When I eat I need to do a blood test and have an injection of insulin. This isn't a problem normally because I only really need to eat at breakfast and lunch and teatime and I can do my blood tests and injections then."

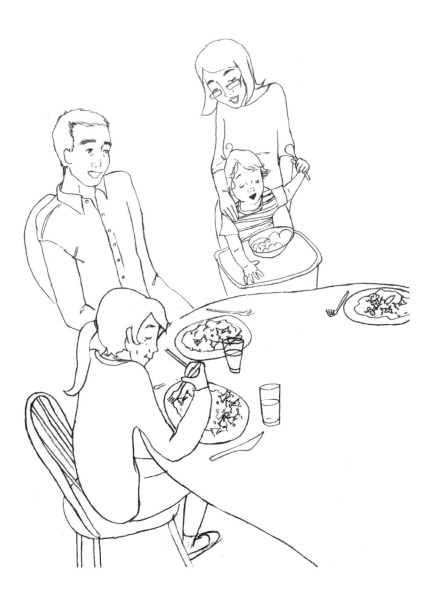

"I can do everything that everyone else
can, but I just need to take time to do some
extra things which I will explain about."

"One of the first things that my grandma said to me when I got diabetes was that I wouldn't be able to eat sweets any more, which made me sad. But it is not true! I can eat whatever I like as long as I know what I am eating and take the right amount of insulin with it.

I have started to learn a lot about food and now I know a lot more than my friends about what is healthy and what is not. I need to eat the same amount of food as all my friends. At first my mum just used to tell me what to eat, but now I have been taught by the dietitian at the hospital how to count the amount of carbohydrate (sugar and starch) in food. This is in foods like bread, potatoes, rice, pasta and cereals, as well as biscuits and sweets."

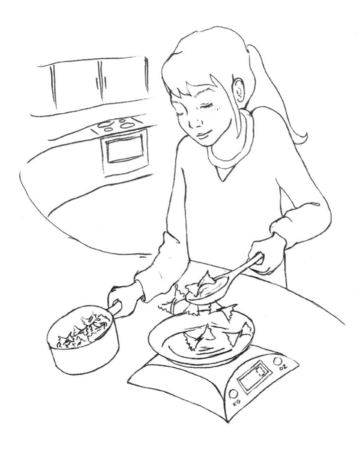

"At every meal or snack, I work out
how much carbohydrate is in the food
I am about to eat, and then I work out
how much insulin to give myself."

"My mum and I have to weigh all the food I eat and work out how much carbohydrate is in it from tables that the dietitian gave us. My friends are getting better at knowing too!

If I want to have a pudding, I have to decide this before I eat so that I can add that carbohydrate into the meal as well and give myself the right amount of insulin for that too, before I start eating.

I use one unit of insulin for every 10 grams of carbohydrate. At lunchtime at school I usually have about 60 grams of carbohydrate (2 slices of thin bread (15 grams in each), a packet of crisps (12 grams) and a small apple (20 grams)). This means that I need to give myself 6 units of insulin just for the food."

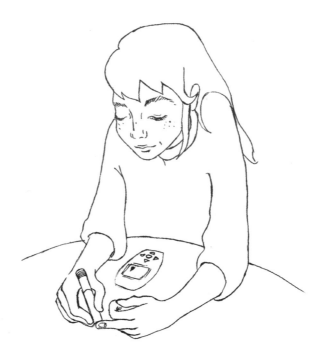

"Before every meal, and when I wake
up and before I go to bed, I have
to prick my finger and use a small
machine to test the drop of blood."

"This is to test the sugar (real name glucose) level in my blood. The level I am aiming for is between 4 and 8 mmol/l (this means millimoles per litre of blood – this is how it is counted).

It is important that I use the side or end of my finger instead of the squishy part in the middle of the end, because I use my fingers for writing and they might start to hurt if I use the wrong bit. I need to use a different finger each time too, or else the fingers will get hard. When I have pricked my finger, I have to squeeze it a bit sometimes (especially if my hands are cold) to make a drop of blood stand up on the finger so that I can get it onto the strip which goes into the blood sugar meter (the machine which measures blood sugar levels). The meter then tells me a number in the little window.

Then I have to lick my finger, or sometimes I wipe it on something like a tissue to stop it bleeding. If I forget to wash my hands before I do the test, the level can be very high, especially if I have been eating something sweet like biscuits and there is still sugar on my hands. That can give me a funny level and I have to do the whole thing again."

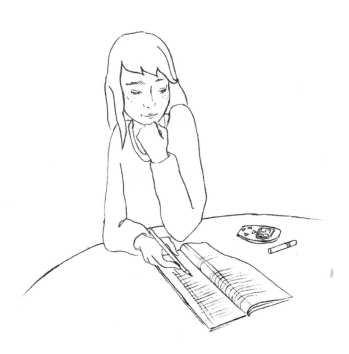

"When I get home I write the blood sugar levels down in a book."

"This means that I can see what has been happening over the past few months and whether the levels are still good. I can talk to my mum if I notice that they are starting to get high.

The blood test before the meal tells me whether my blood sugar is at a good level or not. If it is higher than 8 then I need to add some extra insulin to bring it down to the right level. So I might need more than the 6 units I worked out earlier for my lunch.

The blood meter I have will remember all the levels that I measure for a few weeks, so my parents and I can look back at them to see how things have been going. We can get more information by loading the meter results onto our computer at home and this helps us to decide if we need to change any of the doses I have."

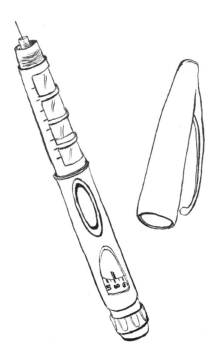

"After I have worked out how much insulin I need, I give myself an injection before every meal or snack."

"I use an insulin 'pen', which looks like a large writing pen. I have to put a needle on to the end of the pen and push a small amount of the insulin out into the air to make sure the needle is full of insulin. At the top end of the pen there is a dial with numbers on and I have to turn it until it shows the right number of units.

I am then ready to inject it. It goes into the thin layer of fat just underneath my skin. This can be done in my tummy or in the top part of my leg (thigh) or the top part of my arm. I think it is easier to do it in my tummy when I am at school because then I don't have to roll down my trousers or roll up my sleeve. I usually sit down to do it and I pinch together some of the skin next to my belly button and do the injection in there."

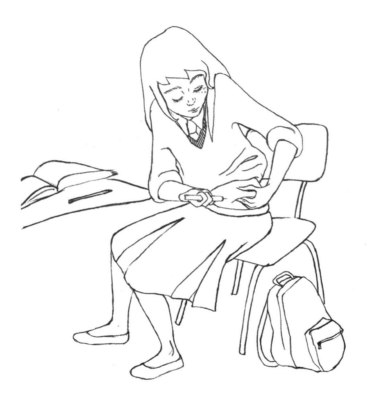

"The injections don't hurt because
the needle is so small."

"Having to remember to do it can be annoying just because the diabetes makes me different from everyone else. My friends understand though, and they usually help me remember to do it before lunch.

I go to the medical room where one of the teachers keeps an eye on me, which I like because it feels private and safe. I know that when I get older I will feel happier doing it in other places like my form room or even in the dinner queue. One of my friends often comes with me too.

The type of insulin I give for my meals is quick-acting insulin because it uses up the food that I eat so that I can keep my blood sugar steady. At home I have a long-acting insulin, which I use just at night before I go to bed. This one lasts all day in between the food insulin. It can sting a bit sometimes, but I have got used to it now."

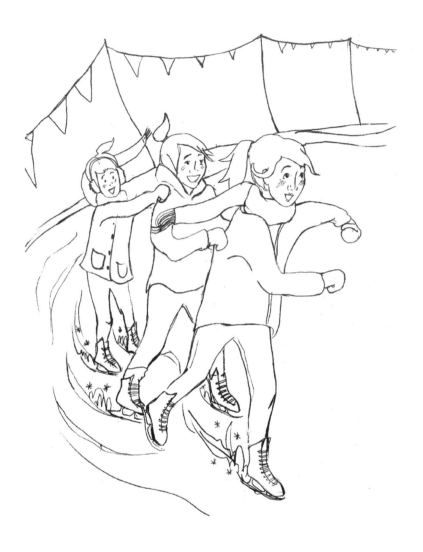

"The other thing that can make a big difference to my blood sugar levels is sport. I am really sporty and play football and hockey and I go ice-skating every week."

"This isn't a problem with my diabetes, but we need to check blood sugar levels more often than usual. I know what I need to eat, and how much insulin to give to make sure that my blood sugar doesn't get too low or too high.

My muscles work best if my blood sugar is about right, and I can usually tell if I am not doing so well at the sport. If I am doing PE at school, my teachers need to know what they should do if my blood sugar goes a bit low, which it might do because I use up energy in my body when I exercise. I drink a sports drink to stop this happening and I don't usually have a problem. Later I will explain what to do if someone you know has low blood sugar."

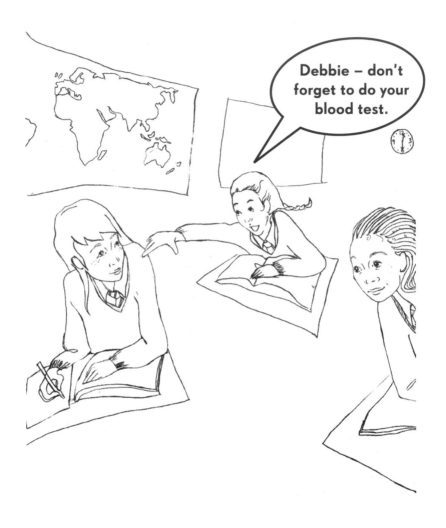

"Generally, having diabetes is not too bad.
But sometimes it is a nuisance and it can be
hard being different from everybody else."

"I don't ever have a day off from it and I have to think all the time about how my food and exercise will affect my blood sugar levels.

I don't like doing my injections when I am out with my family for a meal, because of the way some people look at me. Sometimes I can do it under the table so no one notices, but sometimes I go to the toilet to do it.

People at school have sometimes pretended to be scared of needles or said mean things. They don't always understand how important it is for me to have my insulin. If I didn't get all my injections I would get very sick and ill and could end up in hospital.

Because I understand a lot more than other people about food, I am likely to eat more healthily and do more exercise, which will do me good in the end.

Sometimes I tell people that I have diabetes and they say I must have eaten too much chocolate to get it. I know they are thinking of type 2 diabetes, which sometimes happens when people are overweight, but type 1 diabetes doesn't happen because of this. Most people haven't even heard of type 1 diabetes, even though it is the commonest sort in children."

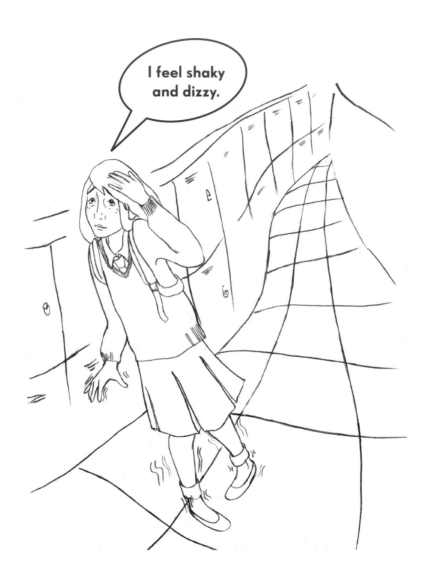

"The level of sugar in my blood can
make a big difference to how I feel."

"I can be grumpy and cross at times, just like anyone else, but sometimes it is because my blood sugar level is high or low.

I had a problem last week. I had given myself an insulin injection at lunchtime but we had to go and work on the school play before I had finished all my lunch. Because I hadn't eaten enough food for the insulin, my blood sugar level went very low.

That usually makes me feel very 'wobbly' and shaky, and sweaty and hungry, but this time I didn't really notice. My friends saw that I wasn't talking properly and wasn't making sense, and looked very pale. They told the teacher and luckily he realised what was going on and let them give me a sugary drink straightaway in the classroom. That made me feel a lot better after about ten minutes and then I had a couple of biscuits and felt as right as rain and could concentrate again.

These low blood sugar levels are sometimes called a 'hypo'. This is from ancient Greek and the full word is hypoglycaemia, which means low (hypo) blood sugar in the blood (glycaemia). The way I feel when I am low or hypo is the way that lots of people feel when they are very hungry, only ten times worse. My hands can get shaky and I feel very wobbly in my legs, and people say I look pale and tired. I can stop concentrating and might start to talk in a strange way and say odd things."

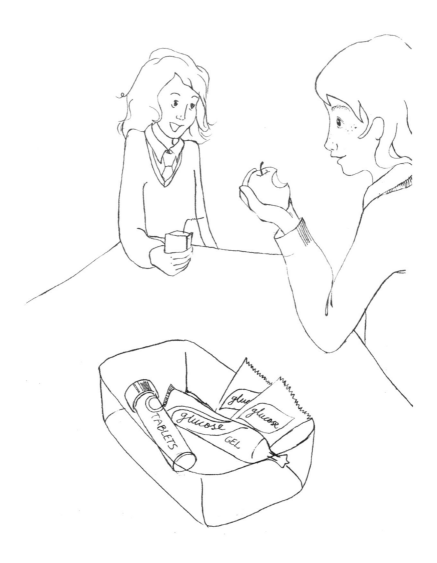

"My nurse says I must do blood tests and be able to eat and drink in the classroom, or wherever I am, when I start to feel 'low'."

"If I don't get the sugar I need quickly I can fall down and become unconscious and could even have fits because of low blood sugar.

So it is best if I am not made to go out into the corridor or made to walk across the school to the medical room if I am feeling low because it would be very dangerous. If I do get sent out of the room (I can't have food in the classroom when we are doing science), then I must have a friend to go with me to make sure I am OK, and I need to eat or drink sugar straightaway.

I have a box in my school bag which has a sugary drink and glucose tablets in it so that I can have something sugary immediately to bring my blood sugar up. If I feel not too bad, I do a blood test to check that my blood sugar is definitely low before I have the drink."

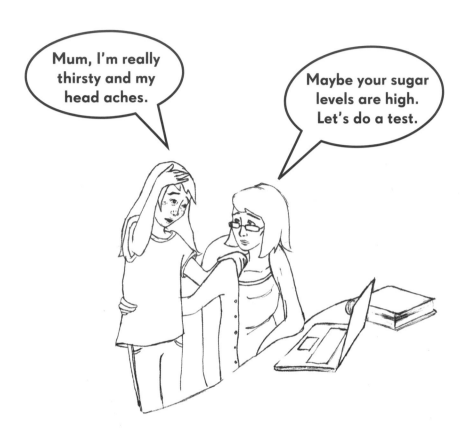

"If I forget to give myself an injection
or if I have a cold or flu I can get
high blood sugar levels."

"A high blood sugar level makes me feel thirsty and can give me a headache. My mum says that I get very 'ratty' at those times and can be quite grumpy with people. I need to do more tests than usual and may need to give myself insulin at odd times, not just when I am eating.

When my blood sugar is high I also need to check my blood for things called 'ketones'. My body makes these when there isn't enough insulin around in my blood. Ketones can make me feel sick, so they are not nice, and I need to give myself extra insulin to get rid of them. But this needs an extra blood test!"

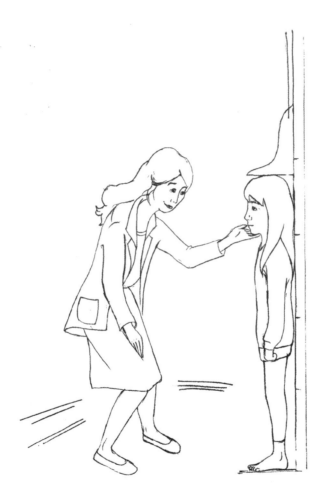

"Every three months I have to go to
the hospital to see my diabetes team.
I always see a doctor and a nurse
and sometimes see the dietitian."

"At the hospital I get measured and weighed, to check that I am growing well. If I didn't have enough insulin, Jane, my diabetes specialist nurse, says I wouldn't grow properly.

At the clinic I have a different finger-prick test which tells me and my mum and dad what my blood sugar levels have been like over the last three months. This helps everyone to know whether I am keeping my diabetes under control.

I then go in and see the doctor and Jane in a clinic room and we chat about how things have been for me. They look at my blood meter and my record book, and will also usually load my meter onto the computer so that we can all have a look at it in the clinic room."

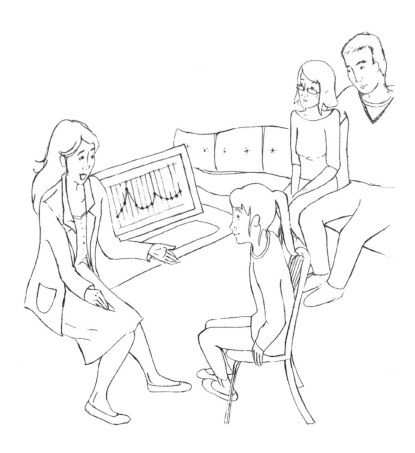

"I can talk to the doctor about what it
is like having diabetes in my life."

"We talk about whether we need to change the amount of insulin I give myself in my injections. The last time I went we also talked a bit about the possibility of me using an insulin pump in the future, instead of injections (more about this later).

Once a year I have to have a proper blood test from my arm. This is to test for other problems that can sometimes happen in people who have type 1 diabetes. I also have to have my eyes tested now that I am over 12, and I have to do some wee (urine) tests as well. These test for protein in my urine and make sure that my kidneys are working fine. The tests have always been OK.

When I was younger I used to kick and scream about the blood test, because I was really frightened of it. I saw a doctor called a psychologist who helped me to cope with my fear of blood tests, and now I can manage to have them done once a year, but I still don't like them!

Sometimes the psychologist is in the room with the doctor and the nurse, and we can just talk about any other problems that I am having. A psychologist is someone who is trained to help children talk about their worries, and who can help them to deal with them. I know that I could talk to the psychologist if I had any other worries about my diabetes."

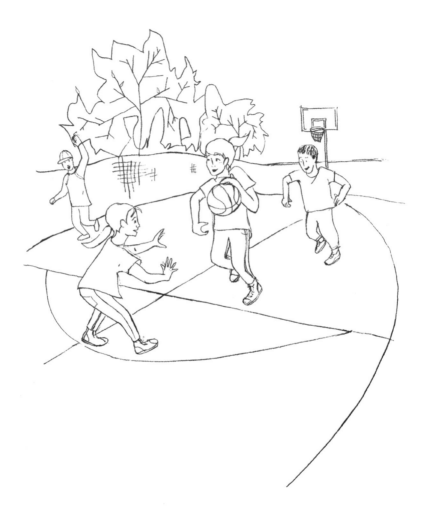

"When I went on an activity weekend with
the diabetes team from the hospital I met
lots of other children with diabetes."

"I had not met any other children with diabetes before, apart from at the hospital, and then we don't usually talk to each other. It was great to meet and talk to other people with diabetes. I have kept in touch with some of my new friends and we can talk about what it is like to have diabetes, which even my parents don't really understand. Some of the other children were using insulin pumps.

My nurse and dietitian also organise teaching sessions for us every couple of years or so. These are extra meetings where we get to talk to other children with diabetes and spend some time (a couple of hours or a half-day) learning about diabetes and how to look after it. I really enjoy these sessions. At the last one we learned about how to count the carbohydrate again and what to do if our blood sugar levels are high when we are ill.

The psychologist was also there and we got into smaller groups to talk about how we would explain that we have diabetes to someone new. That was really helpful because I have just changed school and have had to work out how to look after my diabetes and talk to new friends about it, which has been a bit scary."

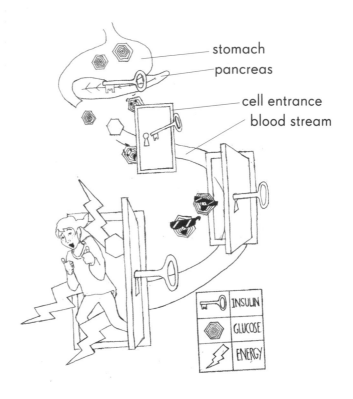

stomach
pancreas
cell entrance
blood stream

🔑	INSULIN
⬡	GLUCOSE
⚡	ENERGY

"In type 1 diabetes, your pancreas, which
is a gland at the back of your tummy,
stops making insulin because it has
stopped working properly. Insulin is made
by the pancreas and moves around your
body making sure that glucose (sugar)
can be used by all the cells in your body
to work properly. If there is no insulin,
the glucose can't get into the cells."

"My specialist diabetes nurse, Jane, explained to me that type 1 diabetes is something that happens in only one in every 400 children in this country. It means that my blood glucose (sugar) levels will get very high and I could be ill and end up in hospital unless I have insulin injections at least four times a day. There are two types of common diabetes, and a few rare sorts.

So, I need to give myself the insulin which isn't being made any more in my body. Some medicines can be eaten or drunk, but insulin isn't like that so it has to be injected or it won't work.

No one really knows why some people get type 1 diabetes, but it is becoming more common in children and they are getting it at a younger age than they used to. It is not something you are born with but it usually starts as a child or teenager. You don't even need to have anyone with diabetes in your family and it is not something that you can catch from someone else. It doesn't happen because of anything you eat, and it is not because you are overweight.

Type 2 diabetes is the sort that usually happens in older people and can often be because people are overweight, but not always. This type is often more common in families where other people have type 2 diabetes.

Children are much more likely to have type 1 than type 2. Type 1 always needs insulin injections, but type 2 can be treated with changes to what you eat, or tablets or insulin injections."

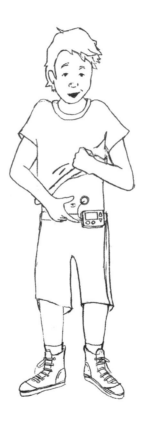

"This is what an injection pump looks like."

"I have told you earlier about my insulin injections. Some people with diabetes don't have injections, but they use an insulin pump. The pump gives them insulin all the time through a plastic tube that goes into a little plastic needle which sits in the thin layer of fat under the skin in their tummy or leg. They can then give insulin just by pressing a button instead of using a needle every time.

This suits some people but I didn't want one of these because of my sport and because I don't want to always be attached to something. I might think about using it in the next year or two though. The pump is just another way of giving yourself insulin, so people who use one still have to do all the other things that I do, like the blood tests and thinking about the food they eat."

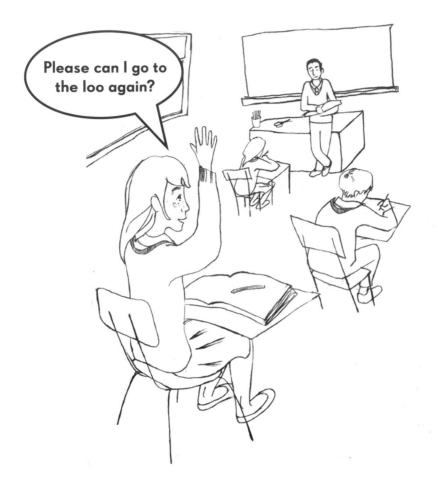

"My parents noticed that I started being very thirsty and drinking all the time, and I needed to go to the toilet a lot more often than everyone else. My teachers also noticed this at school."

"When I first got diabetes my parents didn't know what the matter was but at first they thought it was just because the weather was hot. They didn't know about diabetes or what happens to someone who gets it.

Then mum thought I might have an infection because I had started wetting the bed at night too, so she took me to see the doctor. The nurse at the doctor's surgery did a prick of my finger to get a tiny drop of blood out which she put in a little machine to measure my blood sugar level. It was very high and then she told my mum that we had to go to the hospital straightaway.

At the hospital I had some more blood tests and I had to do a wee into a bottle, and then the doctors told me and my mum that I had type 1 diabetes. I was feeling very sick at the time and couldn't really concentrate.

We were told that it was lucky that my mum had taken me to the doctor when I was still quite well because if you leave it and don't do anything, diabetes can make you very ill. "

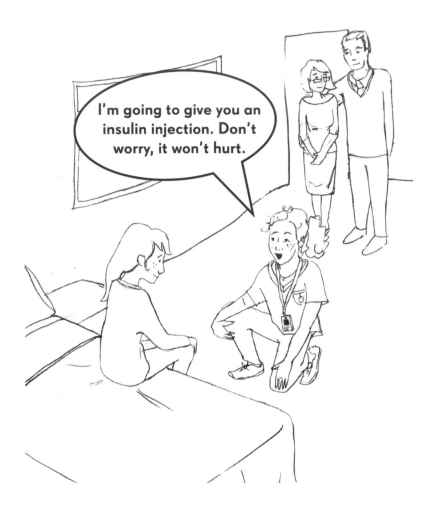

"I was given an injection of insulin with a small needle in my leg. I was very worried that it would hurt at first, but actually I hardly felt it because the needles are so small. And you soon get used to the finger-pricks."

"The nurses had to prick my fingers before all my meals to check my blood sugar level. It was very high to start with and I also had something called ketones in my blood which made me feel sick. But once I started having the insulin, the blood sugar levels gradually came down. And then I started to feel a lot better.

My mum and dad had practised doing the injections and the blood tests in the hospital, so they just carried on doing them when I came home.

My diabetes specialist nurse came out to our house to visit us the day after we got home to check that we were all doing it right and that I was feeling OK. I even went back to school the next week. The nurse had talked to my teachers who helped me with my blood test and insulin injection at lunchtime.

As soon as I felt better, I stopped drinking a lot and going to the toilet all the time. Now I am used to having diabetes."

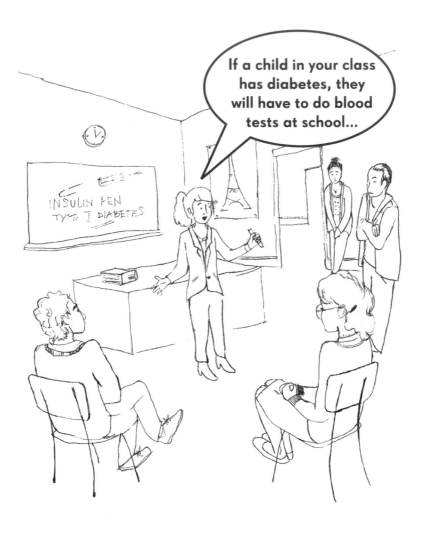

"The headteacher arranged for Jane to visit one lunchtime to help the teachers understand more about diabetes."

"After the talk with the headteacher and my form teacher, I am now allowed to carry my blood meter and some glucose tablets around with me, and there is a sugary drink in a box in the classroom cupboard.

Since diabetes has been explained properly to them, my classmates understand why I have to do different things at lunchtimes and before sport.

Nurse Jane asks how I manage my diabetes at school when she sees me.

I'm so much happier at school now and so my blood sugar levels are better and I can concentrate more and my schoolwork has improved."

How friends can help

- "I am just like everyone else except that my body doesn't make insulin like yours does, and so I need to inject it.

- Sometimes I feel that I don't want to be different and so I try to avoid doing anything about my diabetes. Please let me know that you don't mind if I do an injection.

- Please be patient and wait for me if I have to do a blood test or an injection before a meal or a snack or if we are out together.

- It would help if you could remind me to do the test and injection so that I don't forget.

- If I start to look pale or shaky or I seem not to be concentrating, my blood sugar level might be low. You could ask me to do a blood sugar test to check. Or, if I don't seem to be quite 'with it', just give me a sugary drink. There should be one in my bag or a teacher will know where to find one.

- If I am unconscious, then please lay me on my side while you get adult help.

- Otherwise, please just treat me the same as you would any of your other friends.

- I can still come round for sleepovers and for tea
  like everyone else. My mum will need to be in touch
  with your mum to talk to her about how to look
  after my diabetes."

How teachers can help

"I am happy at school now, but I can still remember the way I used to feel and how frightening it was. Well, that's all changed now, but it may still happen to someone else unless teachers understand more about diabetes and the feelings and worries of children with diabetes. I think it would be brilliant if all teachers could have diabetes training, so they understand more about it. My mum looked up some useful information about school diabetes policies.

- Every school should have a policy to help children with diabetes.

- All of the teachers and staff should be aware of the diabetes policy.

- Schools should also have someone who can help a child with blood tests and injections, especially if they are at primary school or nursery.

In school the best advice to help children with diabetes is:

- If I am not concentrating or being 'naughty' I might have a low blood sugar level. Please ask me to check or do it for me. If I am not quite 'with it', please just give me my sugary drink.

- Make sure my blood testing kit and hypo treatment are easily accessible in the classroom or – even better – that I keep them with me.

- Don't make me leave the classroom to do a blood test or to have some sugar if I need to. It is important that I do it *now* and it would be dangerous to leave me on my own in case my blood sugar level is low.

- Allow me to keep a spare insulin pen in a fridge at school in case the insulin pen I am using runs out or gets broken.

- It would also be nice to have a 'quiet area' at school where I could sit and have my injection at lunchtime, maybe in the medical room or in a school office.

- Allow me to do an extra blood test and eat a snack if necessary to keep my blood sugar level steady before PE.

- It would be great if you could talk to me about diabetes and ask me questions about what will help. I will then feel I can tell you about any problems or fears.

- Try to talk to my parents regularly too, so everyone knows what's going on.

- It would be really good also, if you would explain about diabetes to the other children, who may still not fully understand.

- There are so many things that teachers can do to help. Teachers are responsible for our care during the school day and we trust you and rely on you for your support. Be patient with me. Thank you!"

How parents can help

"Mum and Dad, it's great that you have taken the time to find out so much about diabetes. It really helps me. It would be good if you would continue to do the following things.

- Keep updated with websites such as Diabetes UK.

- Make sure that we attend regular diabetes clinics and education sessions when we're invited.

- If I forget, remind me to take my insulin injection whenever I eat.

- If I go to play sport, remind me to check my blood sugar beforehand and take a glucose drink with me.

- Encourage me to play sport. As well as keeping me fit, it will help to keep my heart, bones and digestive system healthy, as well as improving my blood sugar levels.

- Most importantly, by understanding about my diabetes you will be able to help, encourage, reassure and support me. Thank you!"

Recommended reading, organisations and websites

If you would like to find out more about diabetes, here are some useful books, organisations and websites.

BOOKS FOR CHILDREN

Pesterfield, C. (2003) *Diabetes Made Simple: A Kids' Guide to Type 1 Diabetes*. Crawley, West Sussex: Novo Nordisk.

BOOKS FOR PARENTS AND TEENAGERS

Hanas, R. (2012) *Type 1 Diabetes in Children, Adolescents and Young Adults* (fifth edition). Bridgewater: Class Health.

Ward, F. (2009) *No Added Sugar: Growing Up with Type 1 Diabetes*. London: Hammersmith Press Limited.

Besser, R. (2009) *Diabetes Through the Looking Glass: Seeing diabetes from your child's perspective*. Bridgewater: Class Health.

INTERNATIONAL ORGANISATIONS AND WEBSITES

UK

Diabetes UK

Macleod House
10 Parkway
London
NW1 7AA
Tel: 0345 123 2399
Email: info@diabetes.org.uk
Website: www.diabetes.org.uk

Juvenile Diabetes Research Foundation (JDRF)

19 Angel Gate
City Road
London
EC1V 2PT
Tel: 020 7713 2030
Email: info@jdrf.org.uk
Website: www.jdrf.org.uk

Children with Diabetes

www.childrenwithdiabetes.com/uk

Department of Health

Richmond House
79 Whitehall
London
SW1A 2NS
Tel: 020 7210 5952
Website: www.dh.gov.uk/health/contact-dh

USA
American Diabetes Association
Center for Information
1701 North Beauregard Street
Alexandria
VA 22311
Tel: 800 342 2383
Email: AskADA@diabetes.org
Website: www.diabetes.org

Diabetes Public Health Resource
1600 Clifton Road
Atlanta
GA 30333
Tel: 800 232 4636
Website: www.cdc.gov/diabetes

Children with Diabetes
8216 Princeton-Glendale Road
PMB 200 West Chester
OH 45069 1675
Email: info@childrenwithdiabetes.com
Website: www.childrenwithdiabetes.com

Canada
Canadian Diabetes Association
1400–522 University Avenue
Toronto
ON M5G 2R5
Tel: 416 363 3373
Email: info@diabetes.ca
Website: www.diabetes.ca

Australia

Diabetes Australia
GPO Box 3156
Canberra ACT 2601
Tel: 02 6232 3800
Email: admin@diabetesaustralia.com.au
Website: www.diabetesaustralia.com.au

Australian Diabetes Council
Email: info@australiandiabetescouncil.com
Website: www.australiandiabetescouncil.com
www.diabeteskidsandteens.com.au

New Zealand

Diabetes New Zealand
Classic House
Level 7, 15 Murphy Street
PO Box 12441
Thorndon
Wellington
Tel: 0800 342 238
Email: admin@diabetes.org.nz
Website: www.diabetes.org.nz

Diabetes Youth New Zealand
PO Box 56172
Dominion Road
Auckland 1446
Email: contact@diabetesyouth.org.nz
Website: www.diabetesyouth.org.nz

Blank, for your notes

Blank, for your drawings